CHAKRA
ENERGY
MASSAGE

1st American edition 1988
by Lotus Light Publications
P.O. Box 2
Wilmot, WI 53192 USA
The Shangri-La series is published
in cooperation with Schneelöwe Verlagsberatung,
Federal Republic of Germany
Originally published 1988,
© by Schneelöwe Verlagsberatung, Durach
All rights reserved
Cover design and Art Work: Wolfgang Jünemann
Illustrations: Martina Morlok
Translation and editing: Peter Hübner
Editorial supervision: Monika Jünemann
Production: Schneelöwe, Durach-Bechen,
Fed. Rep. of Germany
ISBN 0-941524-83-3

Printed 1988 in the Federal Republic of Germany

Marianne Uhl

CHAKRA ENERGY MASSAGE

**Spiritual evolution
into the Subconscious
through activation
of the energy points of the feet**

LOTUS LIGHT
SHANGRI-LA

Table of Contents

Foreword

With this book the author presents a holistic method of healing designed for the medical professional as well as the interested layperson.

We have all been made aware of the fact that illness is an expression of spiritual disharmony taking place at the subtle level. Foot reflexology is a diagnostic method that provides us with an aproach to the physical and spiritual planes of the body. It is an ideal means of prevention and early recognition, but also very effective as a means of therapy, especially in cases of psychosomatic and chronic illnesses rooted in particularly deep-seated psychic causes that, unfortunately, can rarely be treated effectively by formal methods of medicine.

An additional aspect of this method of healing that I consider very positive is that here we have a means of treatment nearly totally free of secondary effects for the patient. Neither is the physical integrity of the body injured by injections or pins, nor is there any danger of organ burdening through medication. The body is induced to heal itself, which is the most natural method of treatment a doctor can offer his patient.

I would like to take this opportunity to thank my friend and teacher Marianne Uhl for sharing her knowledge with me – gained through long years of work and experience – and thereby adding to the joy I find in my profession and my life.

Munich, March 1988
Hetty Weber, M.D.

Introduction

Before my dearest and oldest friend and associate Hanne Grym and I began to work out the concept for this book in conjunction with Dr. Hetty Weber, the young "doctor of the future", we first consulted the "Book of Changes"*. It answered our question regarding working on this book with "The Duration".

Specifically it says, "You augment each other fabulously... Your partnership is founded on high and lasting values." As always, the I Ching was right, and I thank both of my friends for the wonderful, harmonious cooperation that led to the creation of this book.

I am also especially grateful to Heike Kletzander, who fulfills her mission of being a catalyst on this Earth for spiritual work so outstandingly, and I thank Inge Helfrich and Jacqueline Theelen for cheerfully taking upon themselves the arduous task of realizing my manuscript.

---

*Quoted from "I CHING – New Systems, Methods and Revelations", Angelika Hoefler, Lotus Light Publications/Shangri-La, 1988.

Our sons Michael and Ulf showed laudible understanding for the fact that their mothers were often not available, and my gratitude also goes to the co-workers at our institute, Renate Adolph and my sister Hannelore Alt, for bearing our frequent absences.

Dr. and Mrs. Simon and Susie Weber generously placed their holiday apartment in a beautiful region of Germany at our disposal, and the peace and positive vibrations there greatly enhanced our work on the book. Heartfelt thanks to them, too.

Monika and Wolfgang Jünemann immediately understood the significance of my work on a spiritual plane and spontaneously supported it. To them and all others that had any part in the realization of this book, I direct my loving thoughts.

My deepest gratitude, however, extends into the spiritual world, to my Masters and Spiritual Guides!

Frankfurt, April 1988
Marianne Uhl

Part I
Fundamentals

Basics of Foot
Reflexology Massage

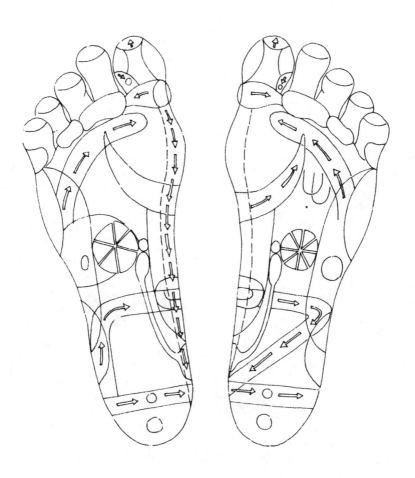

*"When one holds a person's feet
in one's hand, one has hold of
his soul."*

Introduction to Foot Reflexology Massage

The quote at the beginning of this chapter became the foundation of my work. In the course of years of working for and with people, the realization firmed in me that I could not only achieve healing of physical ills using my method of Foot Reflexology Massage, I could also gain deep insight into a person's soul.

I am sure that you are acquainted with foot reflexology as an alternative method of healing. Its effects, however, go far beyond what is commonly known about them, they work much deeper and extend a great deal further...

Sickness is always a physical expression of spiritual discord, which can also be dealt with on the subtle plane. The seven chakras, the body's energy fields, permit us an approach to this plane. They are the links between the physical body, the astral body and the causal realm. The chakras are the connection between the energy body and the physical body. The term "chakra" originates in the Hinduistic Yoga teachings, where the chakras are also connected with the Kundalini-Force via the spine. The energetic quality of the chakras that we are able to feel with our hands is purely subtle vibration. It is the source of our life energy. The astral body is the vibration of our energy body, with which we can leave our physical body. In this way we are connected to the "silver cord" and through it can advance into worlds that no longer contain the limitations of time and space.

The causal realm represents our connection with the Divine. There we share in the cosmic wholeness that is the source of all human beings. On this plane primal knowledge is available to us, that which C.G. Jung defined as the "collective subconscious".

A method of treatment, therefore, that is capable of influencing chakra energy and bringing it into harmony, does not merely treat the symptoms of a physical illness or a phychic disorder, but instead touches upon the real core of the sickness, the "root" of discord.

Precisely this is what we achieve with Chakra Energy Massage. Due to my experience of many years I am well aware of the fact that it can be confusing initially to sort out for oneself the seemingly complex system of Foot Reflexology Massage zones. For this reason I am starting off with an introduction to the fundamentals of Foot Reflexology Massage before presenting the actual work with chakra energy.

No artist will realize his goals if he is not

properly equipped for the task. This means that without fundamental knowledge of Foot Reflexology Massage a Chakra Energy Massage would be ineffective and, in fact, irresponsible.

Therefore my request to you is to take the time to thoroughly read the following pages before you enter into the fascinating world of work with the chakras.

If you decide to embark upon this journey into the subconscious, and do so sincerely and honestly, I assure you that you will discover and experience totally new emotional levels – in yourself as well as in the people to whom you apply this technique.

In harmonizing the chakra energy fields, a positive alteration of consciousness also takes place. Initially it will hardly be discernible, but your perception of your environment and all of your interpersonal relationships will change fundamentally. In your new and harmonious realm of vibration you will not only be freed of illness and disharmonies of body and soul, but will additionally experience new qualities of peace and love in all of creation.

Once having gained this new consciousness you will discover that you are able to enter into meditation, find inner calmness, far more quickly than ever before. You will also be in closer touch with your dreams – our nightly messages for the day to come – and will be able to unfold your healing powers for everyday activities, to activate the healing powers of minerals, fragrances, colors and sounds and even to enter upon astral journeys. In other words, you will be living in harmony with cosmic vibration in all three of your bodies!

Perhaps you are now thinking, "Oh, I know about foot reflexology. A lot of masseurs already use it. This is supposed to be esoteric?"

But please ask yourself if you really know what reflexology zones are and how they function.

Reflexology zones are the terminal points or endings of nerves, and are directly connected to a distant organ or part of the body. Reflexive action of the nervous system that transmits the impulses of all stimuli takes place within the entire body, but the terminal points are located only in the feet.

Dr. Fitzgerald, an American, in 1930 brought forth scientific proof of the so-called "zone therapy", and in doing so discovered ten vertical and ten horizontal nerve fascicles corresponding to the two axes of the body.

For Eunice Ingham, an American masseuse, these facts were the final confirmation of her own observations that in the method of treatment rediscovered by her (a form of a method of acupressure known to have been employed by ancient cultures), the terminal nerve points that could be influenced were located solely in the feet. On the basis of this she was able to further develop Foot Reflexology Massage.

What do we find at the terminal points of the reflex zones?

Within the feet one can feel deposits, also called gravel, consisting of uric acid crystals and other waste products. These are perceptible as hardenings at the terminal points within the reflex zones. In the course of precise palpation, or examining by feeling, these deposits may call forth acute pain and produce light to dark red discoloration. In especially pronounced deposits of uric acid, crystals the size of pin-heads can be felt, and in extreme cases blisters may even appear.

How are these irregularities caused?

Illnesses that are not completely healed by the body's immune system leave their traces in the corresponding reflex zone. Insufficient functioning of the organs involved in eliminating body wastes (kidneys, intestines, lungs and skin) may also cause the depositing of remaining metabolic waste products.

Following treatment by medication we frequently find pharmaceutical residue in the blood and in all of the body's cells, which may form deposits in the manner of the organic waste at the nerves' terminal points, and this particularly often in close proximity to the spinal column.

All of the illnesses a person has experienced since the moment of birth can be determined by the reflex zone terminal points, as most states of sickness are no longer cured naturally, but instead are immediately suppressed by medication.

Chronic illnesses are also caused by this type of treatment and the mechanisms set in motion by it. Additionally, chronic illnesses may be nearly impossible to cure completely, because they are based on a negative thought pattern of which the patient is usually not aware, and which therefore cannot be altered.

Pain in itself is not a disease but instead the clearest possible sign that somewhere within ourselves a part of our body is experiencing a disturbance. The body has no means other than pain to direct our attention to itself. Rather than being negative, pain is therefore a blessing of nature. It is a cry for help! And this is how the initial discomfort and pain that may accompany foot reflexology treatment should be seen.

In our modern times we hardly ever experience natural stimulation of the reflex zones of our feet. Our life environment does not have us walking and running along bumpy roads and accross naturally uneven ground. Today, everything is steamrolled flat, paved and as even as we can make it. We ourselves see to it that the natural circulation in our feet is impaired by wearing cramping foot-gear and synthetic materials. Not only do we spend time in cages – our feet do, too.

Foot reflexology treatment is surely not a cure-all at this time, because "wholeness" requires that a change of consciousness have taken place, which not everyone is prepared to perceive and to realize on his or her own.

As long as this ideal state of wholeness is not yet reached, we will need to interconnect various methods of treatment. Above all we should seek cooperation with medical professionals using natural means of treatment and with non-medical practitioners.

The Chakra Energy Massage represents a chance of attaining this ideal state, because it works a change in our negative, illness-causing thought patterns. Every thought, whether positive or negative, has "vibration" as its original state. Vibrations alone transmit information and make communication possible. And as the chakras are in fact "vibration transformers", a positive modification of vibration quality will necessarily lead to a changing of negative thought patterns. When this relationship has been recognized, one realizes that all thoughts, negative as well as positive, will become manifest. Therefore everyone is fully responsible not only for his or her actions, but also for each single thought!

An old Chinese proverb says, in effect, "Every sickness is a wrong thought. We need only think right, and we will be healthy."

The Massage Technique

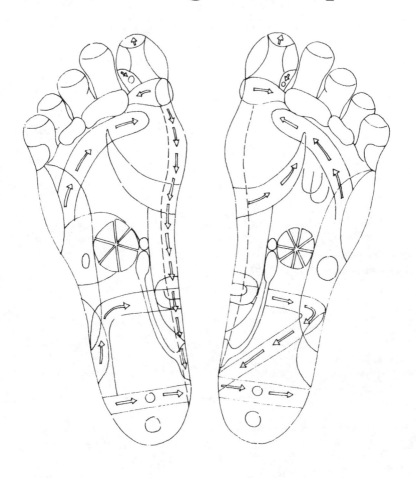

"It is worthwhile, indeed, to take something heavy upon oneself, if in doing so one can ease someone else's burden."

Stefan Zweig

Conducting the Massage

Prior to every massage the terminal nerve points of the feet have to be palpated, i.e. examined precisely by feeling them. This analysis of the terminal nerve points is the prerequisite for effective, purposeful treatment, for it is our only means of determining all of the areas of disturbance present in the body. But this exact palpation is not part of the massage treatment; it is merely acquainting oneself with existing areas of disturbance or waste product deposits.

The procedure is as follows:

Make sure that the patient is resting comfortably, the feet slightly raised. The solar plexus (about one hand's breadth above the navel) should not be cramped, as this would prevent the breath from flowing freely and would impair the function of the autonomic nervous system.

The precise palpation we will require about an hour. The patient's feet should rest on a towel, and it is advisable to have a cream or lotion available to enhance the movement of the hands on the patient's feet. In my own practise I have found a neutral everyday lotion to work best, but whatever you use, please avoid creams or oils that will clog the pores.

After all, the skin is our largest breathing surface. Beyond this we should have a note pad and a pen or pencil at hand.

Moisten your thumbs with lotion or cream and place them in the center of the soles of the feet. Begin the examination by having your thumbs rotate in circular motion (see illustration). Generally, it is easier on the therapist's thumb joints to begin by making larger circles that slowly contract and work their way towards the center of the area. If, however, rotating your thumbs from the center outward feels more harmonious to you, this is just as acceptable.

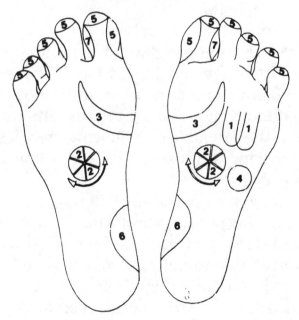

Begin the examination at the solar plexus point with circular thumb movements.

The reflex zone of the solar plexus is the key to our autonomic nervous system and our subconscious. That is why we begin every treatment at this acupressure point. Stabilizing the solar plexus point, which I call "our life's garbage pail", oftentimes results in an immediate loosening of the entire organ area. When pronounced hardening, gravel or cramping are evident here, a patient may occasionally react with violent fits of weeping. This is a "letting go" within the autonomic realm. And don't forget that men are allowed to cry, too!

If such a situation occurs, provide the other person the opportunity to really weep it all out, to experience feelings long suppressed, to permit everything to happen. Crying like this will cease by itself within a few minutes, but you must not interrupt the massage while it is going on. It is a situation you, too, have to bear and go through.

Foot reflexology treatment at the solar plexus point enables one to loosen cramps (blockades) of all sorts besetting body, spirit and soul.

If at this point serious hardening or reddish discoloration become evident, you will have to extend the massage from the usual two minute duration to five minutes. By then the patient will have "let go" sufficiently for you to go on with the step-by-step examination of the other points.

You should always keep in mind that the reflex zone pathways cross at one junction: exactly at the solar plexus. In practise this means that if, for instance, you have localized an indication on the left foot, the disturbance connected with it will be located in the right side of the body, and vice versa.

Only four organs deviate from this principle by conducting directly to the other side without crossing the junction. They are: heart and spleen at the left foot, and liver and gall-bladder at the right foot. (The exact locations of these points are included in the Massage Instructions).

The other single organs and organ systems of the body, such as the spinal column, stomach, uterus, prostate gland, pituitary gland and thyroid gland are aligned with the vertical body axis. They therefore radiate into both sides of the body and have reflex zones in both feet which are, as in the case of organs occurring in pairs, side-inverted.

You are best advised to proceed systematically according to the Massage Instructions and to make note of the terminal points where you were able to determine disturbances. You will soon develop a feeling for discovering significant deposits and spotting discolorations. It is a good idea to make note of these right away, as you will require this information later in order to work out the specific massage program.

The appearance of red discoloration on a foot is in no way related to the duration or intensity of thumb pressure during palpation. If the body is beset by an acute illness, the corresponding zone of the foot will redden immediately.

Do not be afraid of defensive reactions on the part of your patient (after all, nobody is going to permit his inner depths to be looked into just like that!). Make sure that the patient understands that you are the therapist and are taking the responsibility for everything that you are doing. This will help establish a relationship of mutual trust between you, which is the foundation of every healing process, but also the most vital requirement for working with chakra energies.

I would also like to strengthen your self-confidence by assuring you of this: There is nothing that you can do "wrong" when applying this method of massage, and there is no way for you to possibly harm your patient. On the contrary, you are capable of placing the key to his or her body and subconscious in a person's hand – but using it to open the lock is up to each individual alone.

In order to gain a complete picture of the body's state of health you will naturally have to have examined all of the terminal nerve points of the feet at least once. In practise this means that you will start with the left foot and examine the area of the upper head, then immediately take the other foot and do the same. It is most important to always switch from one foot to the other, work down from the toes to the heel, in order to prevent an energy congestion from occurring in the body.

Once you have examined all of the terminal nerve points from top to bottom and have noted your findings, the indications that you have discovered will have to be fitted into the massage guidelines beginning on page 43. It will be best to sort out the notes that you made in the course of the examination in accordance with the three massage programs shown (the Skeletal Program, Digestive Program and Lymphatic Program). This will enable you to determine right away where the emphasis for a given patient of yours should be set, in other words, which program contains the greatest number of organs indicating disturbances.

This main program, regardless of whether you have determined the Skeletal, Digestive or Lymphatic to be appropriate, is the one according to which initial treatment will be applied. As you proceed, be absolutely certain to heed the patient's biological rhythm. Which is to say, do not massage daily. Massages must always have intervals of at least 24 hours between them in order to give the body time to eliminate waste matter that has been activated.

Also keep in mind that the deciding factor is not how strongly or forceful you conduct the massage, as your hands not only apply pressure, they also transmit warmth and life energy.

In the course of this work, true comunication from body to body and soul to soul takes place.

Time is also an important factor in this program. Reflexology zones with deposits that can be felt but show no reddish discoloration are massaged for approximately two minutes.

Should slight reddening set in, however, extend the massage time for those zones to five minutes.

If an acute condition is obviously given (dark red color or a blister), you should allow seven minutes of massage for those reflex zone terminal points.

Your treatment can be considered a success when reddening no longer sets in, usually after three to seven massage sessions. You can then return to applying two-minute massages.

But please keep one thing in mind:

If serious indications (dark red color or blistering) set in, yet the patient is unaware of corresponding damage to his system or illness, you must see to it that he or she undergoes a medical examination at the hands of a professional utilizing natural means of healing or a non-medical practitioner. Then you should continue massaging only after you have informed yourself regarding the diagnosis and have discussed the matter with the diagnosing professional or practitioner.

Should indications point to a dental problem, the tooth will, of course, be a matter for a dentist. But the area surrounding the roots of a tooth may well benefit from improved circulation and activation through Foot Reflexology Massage, which could thusly enhance the healing process within the jaw area.

If parodontosis or other ailments of the gums are the case, the corresponding reflex zone may be massaged by itself daily, independently of a given massage program. In cases of acute or previous states of parodontosis you may (as a safeguard against recurrance, too) include this reflex zone in any of the programs, regardless of whether you are applying the Skeletal, Digestive or Lymphatic, prior to beginning the closing relaxation phase.

Massage Instructions (short description)

The patient should be lying comfortably. The feet should always be raised a bit, and care taken to insure that the entire body and particularly the solar plexus region are unimpeded and in no way constricted. Have a towel or paper towels at hand, as well as cream or lotion and your notes and the massage program you have prepared.

Every massage begins with the solar plexus points, which are massaged simultaneously on the right and left foot. The rest of the massage is conducted according to the program you have decided on, whereby you continue along the soles and, if indicated, along the sides and tops of the feet all the way to the heels. Without exception massages are brought to a close with the Relaxation Program – by exerting gentle pressure on the lymphatic area. The arrows in the illustrations indicate the direction in which you can massage so that the pressure of your rotating thumb always tends to move towards the center.

Massage Instructions:
Soles of the feet

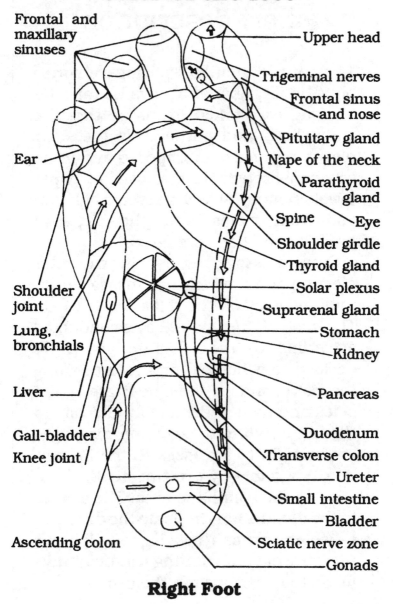

Frontal and maxillary sinuses

Upper head

Trigeminal nerves

Frontal sinus and nose

Pituitary gland

Ear

Nape of the neck

Parathyroid gland

Spine

Eye

Shoulder girdle

Thyroid gland

Shoulder joint

Solar plexus

Suprarenal gland

Lung, bronchials

Stomach

Kidney

Liver

Pancreas

Gall-bladder

Duodenum

Knee joint

Transverse colon

Ureter

Small intestine

Bladder

Ascending colon

Sciatic nerve zone

Gonads

Right Foot

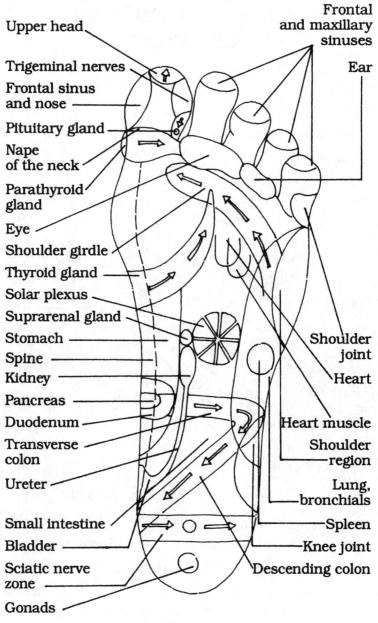

Upper head

Trigeminal nerves

Frontal sinus
and nose

Pituitary gland

Nape
of the neck

Parathyroid
gland

Eye

Shoulder girdle

Thyroid gland

Solar plexus

Suprarenal gland

Stomach

Spine

Kidney

Pancreas

Duodenum

Transverse
colon

Ureter

Small intestine

Bladder

Sciatic nerve
zone

Gonads

Frontal
and maxillary
sinuses

Ear

Shoulder
joint

Heart

Heart muscle

Shoulder
region

Lung,
bronchials

Spleen

Knee joint

Descending colon

Left Foot

37

Massage Instructions: Side View

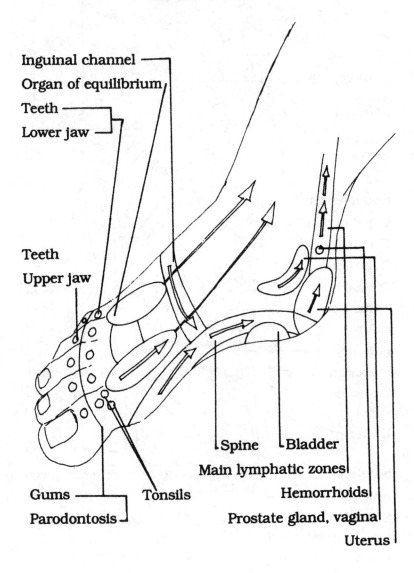

Inguinal channel

Organ of equilibrium

Teeth

Lower jaw

Teeth

Upper jaw

Spine

Main lymphatic zones

Gums

Tonsils

Parodontosis

Hemorrhoids

Prostate gland, vagina

Uterus

Bladder

Right Foot

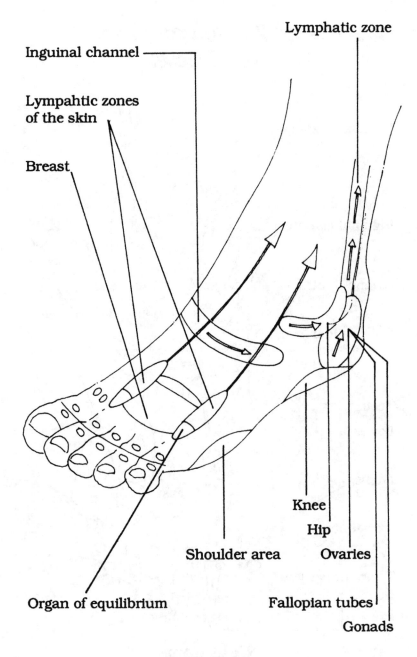

Lymphatic zone

Inguinal channel

Lympahtic zones
of the skin

Breast

Knee

Hip

Shoulder area   Ovaries

Organ of equilibrium   Fallopian tubes

Gonads

Left Foot

39

Massage Instructions: Top View

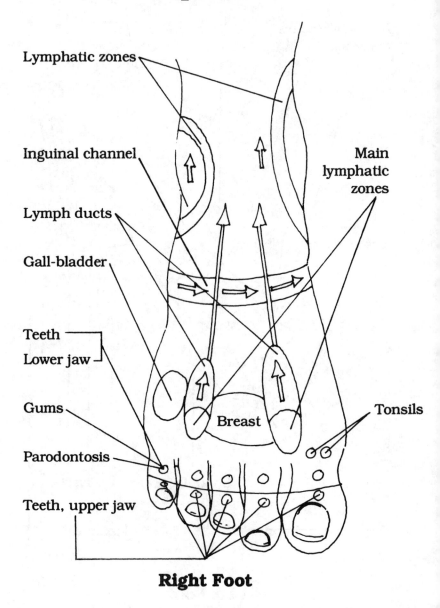

Lymphatic zones

Inguinal channel

Lymph ducts

Gall-bladder

Teeth
Lower jaw

Gums

Parodontosis

Teeth, upper jaw

Main lymphatic zones

Breast

Tonsils

Right Foot

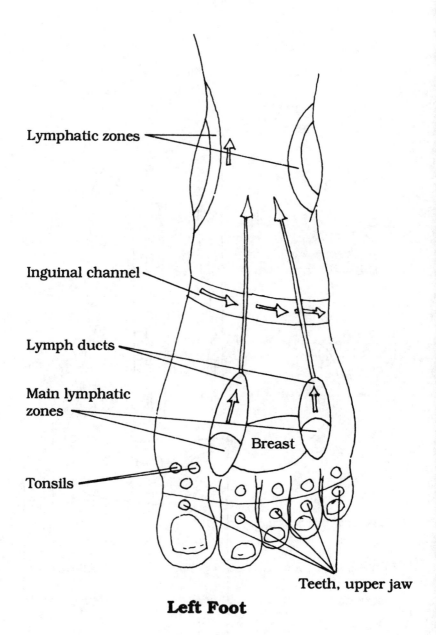

Lymphatic zones

Inguinal channel

Lymph ducts

Main lymphatic zones

Breast

Tonsils

Teeth, upper jaw

Left Foot

Massage Instructions: Heel View

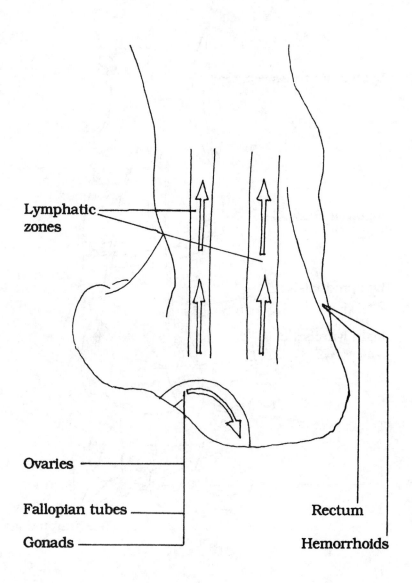

Lymphatic zones

Ovaries

Fallopian tubes

Gonads

Rectum

Hemorrhoids

Guidelines for the Development of Massage Programs

The following massage guidelines are meant to assist you in working out individual massage programs. They will enable you to sort out various indications and changes discovered during your detailed palpation (such as gravel, reddening up to a dark red degree and hardenings), and to class them with the Skeletal Program, Digestive Program or the Lymphatic Program.

Start off the first massage session with the program which contains the largest number of indications that you have noted. The next program may be applied during the following massage session. All three programs are never applied on the same day. Instead, only one program is used during a given session. (And please keep the 24 hour intervals in mind).

Massage Guideline
1. Skeletal Program

Solar plexus
Upper head
Frontal sinus, nose
Maxillary sinus
Trigeminal nerves
Nape of neck, cervical vertebrae
Shoulder joint
Shoulder girdle
Shoulder region
Spinal column
Sciatic nerve
Hip
Knee
Relaxation

Teeth*
Gums*

*May be included in any program if indicated

Massage Guideline
2. Digestive Program

Solar plexus
Heart*
Lungs, bronchials
Liver, gall bladder
Stomach
Kidney, ureter, bladder
Intestine including duodenum
Pancreas and small intestine
Spleen
Heart**
Relaxation

* In case of low blood pressure should be
  massaged following solar plexus

**If high blood pressure is the case, massage prior
  to relaxation

Massage Guideline
3. Lymphatic Program

Solar plexus
Pituitary gland
Parathyroid gland
Ears
Eyes
Thyroid gland
Uterus/prostate gland
Ovaries/gonads
Tonsils
Equilibrium
Chest region
Inguinal channel
Lymph/hemorrhoids
Relaxation

Ending the Massage:

The Relaxation Program

At the end of every massage something lovely and pleasant takes place, sort of a "reward" for possible discomfort or pain that perhaps had to be borne: the relaxation massage.

Patients are usually at a high level of relaxation and detachment as they enjoy the good feelings now being given them. Oftentimes they will visualize images, pictures and wonderful colors. We see this phase as "giving love" with our hands.

You massage without pressure, very lightly and gently, with soft circular motions along the main lymphatic lines on the upper side of the foot towards the ankle (illustration p.48). Let your feeling be your guide as you are doing this, but always begin simultaneously on the outer areas of both feet. Then slowly work your way towards the big toes and almost imperceptibly massage these lymphatic lines, too, in the direction of the ankle. In closing, gently stroke along the tops of both feet several times up beyond the ankle.

Allow yourself at least ten minutes time for the relaxation massage.

This closing massage is also a wonderful

means of harmonizing persons whose autonomic system is beset by pronounced disturbances, so that after being "treated" in this manner for a while, they will be able to permit themselves to undergo usual foot reflexology treatment.

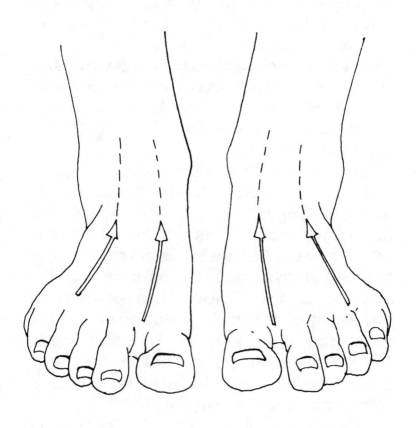

Gently stroke along the tops of the feet

This massage is equally effective as preparation for autogenous training or meditative practise, as it enhances entry into the phase of calmness.

You can simply regard this closing "massage" as a window which one opens in order to let fresh air containing lots of oxygen in.

If your patient has to return into his or her daily routine right after your treatment and will not be able to spend a while in the final, gentle state of "floating", you will have to employ an "awakening" procedure. This is best done by holding the sole of the patient's foot with one hand, making a fist with the other hand, and rolling your fist down along the sole from the toes to the heel.

Part II
The Chakra Energy Massage

The Chakra Energy Massage

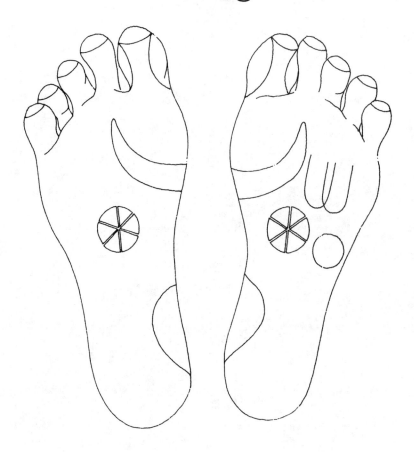

"Only he encounters his limitations, who believes in their existence."

The Progression of Foot Reflexology Massage into Chakra Energy Massage

For many years I practised Foot Reflexology Massage according to the method I briefly presented in the first part of this book. Although spiritual experiences had occurred to me as far back as my early youth, the circumstances of my life were such that I was not yet able to create a synthesis of my daily activities and my spiritual life. It was a very radical personal experience that finally made it possible for me to realize that my work and the other aspects of my life could come into perfect union.

One day in the course of my regular evening meditation it became obvious that I was incapable of achieving inner peace and calmness. I was constantly experiencing visions of organs and parts of the body before my inner eye.

The thyroid gland, uterus, spleen and heart appeared – devoid of any context and making no sense whatsoever.

My inital reaction was to say to myself "You've been working too hard. You'll calm down in due time..."

But after a number of weeks, even after having taken a long, relaxing vacation, my inner peace had still not returned. Visions of organs still forced themselves on me as I meditated. As a matter of fact, my meditative experiences took on increasing intensity. Often I was caught up in regular ecstasy of color. All of this was totally unexplainable to me and I became increasingly worried. I listened for my inner voice and asked my spiritual guide to provide me with the right impulses and to show me what all of this meant, because contrary to my usual way of seeing things, these experiences were becoming more and more uncanny for me. In other words, I had reached a point where I hardly knew myself.

For me there is no such thing as a coincidence, and so I was not particularly surprised when, of all times, it happened in the middle of moving into a new home that the solution to my tortured state of many weeks revealed itself to me.

I was busily cleaning out the basement, packing books and other material from my earlier years of studying into boxes, and my son was there helping me. Then, for some reason, a box fell to the floor and burst open. I had an impatient remark on the tip of my tongue when what I was looking at suddenly stopped me. Scattered before my feet was old material from my days as a trainee, and the uppermost sheet showed the seven chakras, our main energy centers.

I stood there paralyzed!

In a flash I realized where my inner tension had come from. It was totally clear to me at that moment that these were all organs – and the only ones – that I had seen with my inner eye while meditating!

It was as if a fever had taken hold of me. I could hardly get out of that basement fast enough, and from then on packing for our move no longer interested me in the least. Excitedly I searched for the file that contained my tables on foot reflexology, and I hoped desperately that it hadn't been packed yet!

Before my eyes the seven organ systems that physically represent the chakras and the terminal nerve points of the feet, which I had so often touched in the past, united to form one meaningful entity. Now I had comprehended the message sent by the spiritual world:

"The reflexology zones are the spiritual evolution into the subconscious."

And now I also had the explanation for the feelings of dissatisfaction that I often experienced when treating certain patients. It had been proven that organically there was nothing wrong with them, and yet they suffered considerable pain when these points were massaged, which I now recognized to be those of the chakras.

When this occurred I always had the vague feeling that the reflexology zones were trying to tell me more – but up until then I had been unable to understand them.

With this book I would like to pass on to all those interested and searching the knowledge of how really simple it is to dissolve blockades in people, so that a step toward holistic healing may be taken.

In my opinion, neither orthodox medicine nor alternative methods of healing have managed to reach this goal to date.

Although great results have been achieved in specialized areas, the wholeness of the human being, consisting of body, spirit and soul, has always been neglected.

In my own life I have often had to experience pain through personal suffering, and I recognized how frequently my soul was simply forgotten, no matter how well-meaning the doctors and therapists were.

Through the foot reflexology terminal points we are given the wonderful opportunity of not only achieving physical healing by applying Chakra Energy Massage, but to healingly influence the astral and causative bodies as well.

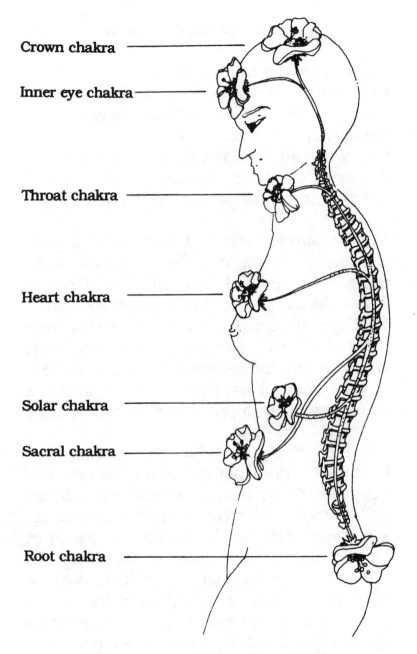

Crown chakra

Inner eye chakra

Throat chakra

Heart chakra

Solar chakra

Sacral chakra

Root chakra

The main human energy centers (chakras)

The seven organs corresponding to the seven chakras:
the heart to the heart chakra
the solar plexus to the solar chakra
the thyroid gland to the throat chakra
the spleen to the sacral chakra
the frontal sinus to the inner eye chakra
the sacrum to the root chakra
the pituitary gland to the crown chakra

On the purely biological level these organs also help regulate important processes connected with the body's metabolism. This explains the popular medical excuse and catchall diagnosis that someone is suffering from "neurodystonia" as actually being a condition of insufficient interaction on the part of these seven organs at the physical level, which is caused by disharmony in the realm of energy on the subtle plane.

In the many cases of people suffering from "instability" and "neurasthenia", where they may even be declared to be hypochondriacs and therefore despair and f eel misunderstood, one will always discover blockades in one or more of the chakras. Applying the Chakra Energy Massage, a relatively simple method of treatment, can literally "free" these people and give them back their belief in themselves, which they have often lost in the course of their search for healing.

After I had recognized the connection between foot reflexology and the chakras, I first tried experiments on myself.

I massaged the chakra points on my feet prior to my meditations. After doing so I managed to enter into the phase of calmness unusually fast. "Letting go" led me further into the depths of my subconscious, and from the spiritual world I received another vision, which is relevant for work with the chakras.

The individual energy fields appeared in total clarity before my inner eye. Each chakra radiated its own special color, as I had never seen it before. But in spite of this they were familiar to me – they were the colors of the human aura.

For people with the gift of seeing auras it is possible to gain something like a "clinical picture" from their radiation. Along with other ills they are capable of identifying blockades, congestions, drainage and even forms of obsession and posession.

Each of these individual colors with its specific vibration corresponds to the vibrations of the chakra, to which it belongs, and in this way can develop healing effects.

At the same time, this vibration is part of a person's sum total of energetic vibrations on the subtle plane. Thus the circle of human wholeness is completed, and the conclusion lies at hand that disturbances within one chakra must necessarily have a detrimental effect on the sensitive vibrations of the aura in its entirety.

Following the transformation of the basic knowledge, in other words, the conversion of knowledge to wisdom by means of messages from the spiritual world and my being permitted to perceive from out of the subconscious, a great feeling of peace spread in me, for I knew now that I was on the right path towards the development of a holistic method of healing. I made my spiritual experiences with colors a part of my new chakra energy program. Thus the colors received their significance as healing forces by being appropriately related to the chakras.

The healing color
of the heart chakra is pink,
of the solar chakra is yellow,
of the throat chakra is blue,
of the sacral chakra is orange,
of the inner eye chakra is violet,
of the root chakra is red and
of the crown chakra is gold.

Just as a prism breaks down sunlight into its spectral colors, so the white gold of the crown chakra, our most spiritual plane, divides itself into the other healing colors.

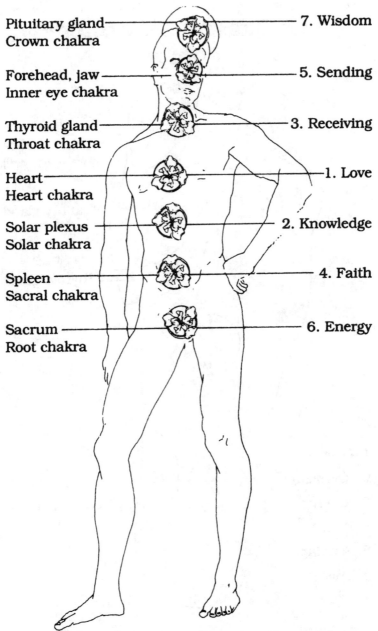

Pituitary gland
Crown chakra

7. Wisdom

Forehead, jaw
Inner eye chakra

5. Sending

Thyroid gland
Throat chakra

3. Receiving

Heart
Heart chakra

1. Love

Solar plexus
Solar chakra

2. Knowledge

Spleen
Sacral chakra

4. Faith

Sacrum
Root chakra

6. Energy

*The chakras, the organs, glands and body parts
relating to them and their spiritual planes*

The Chakra Reflexology Points

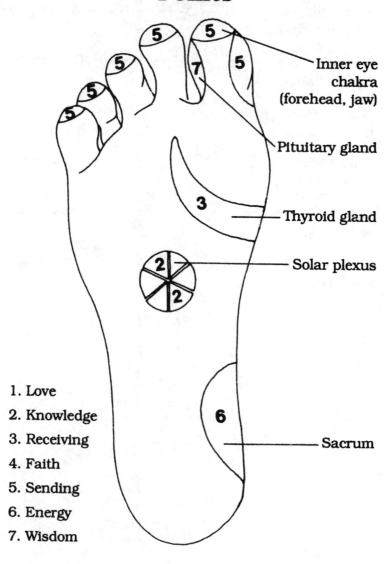

Inner eye chakra (forehead, jaw)

Pituitary gland

Thyroid gland

Solar plexus

Sacrum

1. Love
2. Knowledge
3. Receiving
4. Faith
5. Sending
6. Energy
7. Wisdom

Right Foot

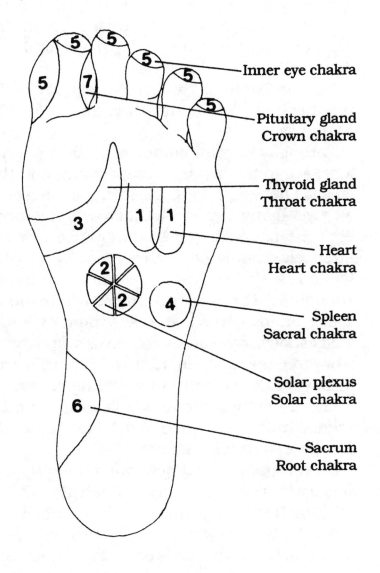

Inner eye chakra

Pituitary gland
Crown chakra

Thyroid gland
Throat chakra

Heart
Heart chakra

Spleen
Sacral chakra

Solar plexus
Solar chakra

Sacrum
Root chakra

Left Foot

65

In the final form of our spiritual development all of the chakras radiate this highest, purest white light clear as diamonds, the most supreme expression of the perfection attained. Then we are truly in harmony and enlightened.

On the basis of this realization very definite healing possibilities then unfold for the therapist.

Through the combination of Chakra Energy Massage in the sense of acupressure and the specific healing colors, which can be presented visually by lamps, cloth, colorful pictures etc., the patient's self-healing processes are intensely stimulated. In this, his active participation is also of great importance. It is not enough for the patient to merely "consume" the colors passively; he or she must by auto-suggestion immerse in the color's sphere of vibration, must open him- or herself completely for the color and its healing power.

Life is always vibration: colors, sounds, scents, minerals, each single atom, all is merely a rotation of energy.

Do you understand now, what the quintessence of Einstein's theory of relativity is?

All matter is vibration – whether visible or invisible. In this way the wholeness of Creation, too, becomes comprehensible for us: the microcosm corresponds completely to the macrocosm, above is below, positive pole is negative pole, inhaling is exhaling and – death is life. For energy is never lost, it is merely transformed into another form of vibration. There is no such thing as death!

With these realizations the present state of my work in foot reflexology within the chakras has matured to completeness.

The vibrations of each single chakra can also be harmonized and intensified through the energy radiation (vibrations) of the corresponding fragrant essences, which I have determined by conscientious testing and experience.

The same applies for the specific sound frequencies which can stimulate their corresponding chakras with extremely subtle vibrations. These sounds are particularly effective with patients that are no longer grounded, that have lost the original frequency of their chakras.

Through the specific application of Chakra Energy Massage, the corresponding colors, healing stones, the appropriate fragrances and especially the so-called "primary tones", one can, in a sense, synchronize the spheres of vibration: the patient returns into harmony with the universal vibration.

All crystals have a singular, subtle energy that they alone posess. Healing stones, on the other hand, have a very special quality that is the reason for their oftentimes astoundingly strong effects. They have frequencies that correspond harmoniously to the chakras and thereby can develop healing effects, in other words, influence the chakras positively.

Can you feel already, what powerful healing effects and possibilities lie in the interconnecting of all of these vibrations?

Stay with me on this continuing journey through each of the chakras.

In my descriptions and analyses so far you may have missed the healing color green, which a number of authors assign the heart chakra.

The fact is that in the course of my spiritual experiences I was never able to establish harmony with green for the heart chakra. Without my wanting it to or being able to do anything about it, the green transformed itself into pink during every heart chakra meditation I have undertaken. By way of an explanation the only thing that occurrs to me is that the green bud of the rose will, as it ripens, irresistably bring forth the pink of the young blossom, and so the true color of the opened heart chakra is a tender pink.

Yet the color green posesses an important therapeutic quality. It is not assigned to any organ, but rather the healing color for the entire body. The suggestive envelopment of the body in green light has a tremendously relaxing and harmonizing effect on the organism as a whole, similar to a long walk through the green aura of woods and meadows. In this way we spiritually utilize the healing powers of the nature that surrounds us.

Before I introduce you to the technique of Chakra Energy Massage, for your personal spiritual development I would like to explain the reason for and the significance of the order in which the chakras are presented:

Contrary to the ususal Foot Reflexology Massage, as presented in the first part of the book, the initial massage now is not performed on the solar plexus zone (the solar chakra), but instead on the zone of the heart chakra. We first open ourselves in the sphere of emotion and unite with all-encompassing love.

In order to then create an equilibrium in the development of the chakras, we now alternatingly activate one of the lower and immediately afterwards one of the higher chakras.

Thus the yin-yang principle remains completely unimpaired and a balance between the physical and the spiritual worlds is maintained.

Next we therefore activate the solar chakra (earth-bound), then the throat chakra (spiritual), then the sacral chakra (earth-bound), followed by the inner eye chakra (spiritual), then enter the power of the root chakra (earth-bound) and take all of this elementary energy up along the spinal column into the crown chakra – our highest spiritual plane.

Only in this manner can elementary driving force be transformed into our genuine life energy. Because we are of this world – and yet are not of this world.

Through my experiences with the power of the chakras I know that it is not advisable to begin with the root chakra, to merely develop energy from below and bring it up, as propagated by various meditation techniques.

Being bound to the Earth is an important component of our incarnation. When we forget this and neglegt to integrate our lower chakras harmoniously, we may "drift off", and then we will not be able to accomplish our mission here on Earth anymore.

As important as spiritual development may be and is, it nevertheless cannot be our sole and single goal. When one withdraws onto an exalted spiritual plane – without having fulfilled one's mission in the Here and Now (the nature of which each of us has to find out personally) – one is fleeing from the real meaning of life and has not fulfilled one's karma.

We will now proceed step by step and develop the activation of each individual chakra. As we do this, please keep in mind the basic rules for resting and treating the patient as explained for Foot Reflexology Massage on pages 27 – 34.

The Heart Chakra

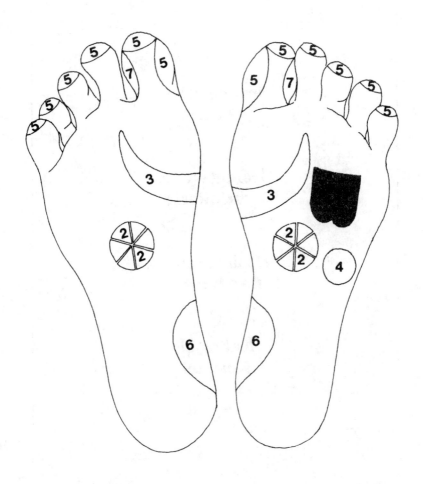

*"There is only one great power
on Earth – and that is love."*

Healing color:
Pink

Healing stone:
Rose quartz

Healing tone:
Earth tone

Healing oil:
Rose oil

Heart Chakra Massage

Ask your patient to first of all visualize his or her heart as the organ it is before his inner eye and to envelop it in warm pink. If the patient finds it difficult to visualize the color, you should make it easier for him or her to conjure it up, for instance by suggesting concentration on a known object that is pink. This often makes initial visualization easier. For you as the therapist this will serve as a first signal that there is a blockade present in this chakra.

Patients frequently complain about functional heart disorders, heart rhythm irregularities, bouts of angina pectoris or high blood pressure for which no organic cause can be determined. Psychosomatically these people are living their loneliness, their inability to find contact – in short, their deficiency of love – as heart disorders in the broadest sense of the word, or they are fleeing into dependency on alcohol, pills or drugs in order not to have to "feel" this lack of love in themselves or in their environment.

Basically, you already know the massage technique from reading the first part of the book:

You begin with the left foot and massage the

terminal nerve point of the heart for two minutes using circular pressure. Here, also, you will be able to feel the indications already described if blockades are there (reddening, swelling, gravel, hardening).

These disturbances will be loosened a lot faster and easier, however, if you utilize the healing effect of the crystal whose vibrations correspond to this chakra energy. I have found time and again that rose quartz posesses the ideal vibration for this and therefore has the strongest healing effect.

There are other stones that have positive influence on the heart chakra, but their healing force is not nearly that of rose quartz. The only mineral that can be employed universally and to a degree may serve as a substitute for any healing stone is rock crystal.

The specific vibrations of rock crystal can enter into contact with the vibrations of all of the chakras and thereby purify, but their effect will not be elementally healing. This explains the positive influence rock crystal has on all of the energy centers.

It is therefore best to place a rose quartz onto the heart area while you are massaging. This will make it easier for the patient to concentrate on the heart. Let the patient feel the stone's vibrations. Trust in it and let the patient do so, also, although he or she may not perceive it at the outset. In the course of the massage but at the latest during the time afterwards, things will begin to change. But many of my patients spontaneously declare that they feel a pleasant pulsing or a warm sensation while they are being treated.

Should you have determined that the person you are treating has a blockade of the heart chakra, you should additionally advise him or her to bring the healing power of the color pink into everyday life. Pink may, for instance, be worn more frequently, or become manifest through deliberately chosen flowers, and thus mobilize the healing power of the color via the subconscious by constantly having it present. The next time the patient comes for a Chakra Energy Massage you might also support your work with pink-colored cloth, flowers and similar means.

The sound frequency correspondimg to the heart chakra is the earth tone. This primary tone is in harmony with the vibrations of the planet Earth – it is the expression of life – synchronous to the biological rhythm of our bodies.

For practical reasons it is hardly possible during a Chakra Energy Massage to employ all of the primary tones in sequence. My advice is, therefore, to simply use meditational music of your choice during the first massage, during which you may be in the process of finding possible indications of blockades.

Once you know where the patient's personal problems and vulnerabilities lie, you can employ a fitting primary tone corresponding to your findings during the next session.

In order to round off the Chakra Energy Massage perfectly I recommend that you employ fragrant essences (essential oils), because we also absorb vibrations with our sense of smell. Particularly scents can make us more permeable for subtle energies, and mere traces that reach our subconscious exercise a strong effect on the human energy body.

The fragrance of the heart chakra is that of the rose. If a patient's heart chakra is blocked, he or she should – prior to every treatment – put a drop of pure rose oil on the location of the inner eye, under the nose and also on the first cervical vertebra, and then inhale deeply three times.

Use this and the fragrances yet to be discussed solely for the blocked chakra in question.

Once you have interconnected all of these vibrations (massage, color, healing stone, tone and fragrance) the chakras will, as time passes, return to their original, harmonious vibrations and form spirals opening towards the top into the causal realm.

Your massage of the heart point should last

about two minutes, after which you let the activated energy field spiritually flow into the SOLAR CHAKRA.

The Solar Chakra

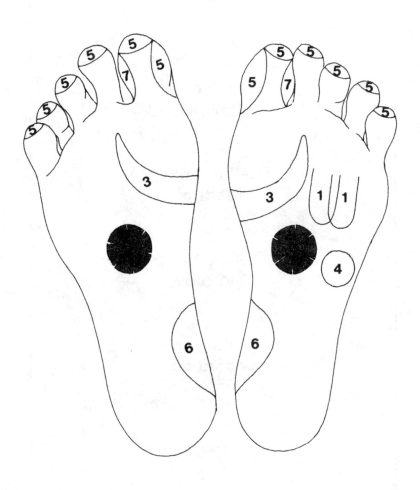

"Carry the Sun in your Heart..."

Healing color:
Yellow

Healing stone:
Citrine

Healing tone:
Sun tone

Healing oil:
Lemon oil

Solar Chakra Massage

Simultaneously take hold of the left and the right foot and again massage the solar plexus point on both feet for two minutes. Here it is important that you have the patient visualize the healing color yellow prior to your beginning with the second chakra. Utilize the same procedure described for the heart chakra.

Most people will have little difficulty visualizing the sun or a sunflower. You will be amazed at the feelings that patients that are concentrating on being within their own abdomen with these visualizations will decribe for you!

The physical manifestation of a disturbance within the solar chakra may take on such diffuse forms as frequent feelings of fullness and a tendency to be constipated, but also serious conditions such as colitis ulcerosa, chronic gastritis or various forms of ulcers.

The solar plexus is the focal point of our primal knowledge and it also reflects all of our fears. We all know what "butterflies in the stomach" feel like. That is our solar plexus reacting.

As I have said previously, the solar chakra is the "garbage pail" of our soul, and for this reason feelings long buried and suppressed will be set free during the Chakra Energy Massage – everything one has "swallowed" in the course of time – and this will frequently be accompanied by violent, yet liberating fits of weeping. When this occurs, by all means let the patient come to grips with his or her pain alone, continue massaging calmly and evenly and do not attempt to quiet or divert the person – they have a right to their own tears.

After a few minutes calmness will set in again by itself and the patient will most likely be exhausted, but feeling unburdened and deeply relaxed. Support the purefying effects of the massage with the healing stone of the solar chakra, the citrine. I have found time and again that its vibrations are an ideal augmentation for this chakra.

When doing so, proceed as described previously, placing the stone a hand's breadth above the patient's navel. The stone's intense warmth will be noticed right away.

You can further enhance your treatment within the solar chakra by employing the sun tone. It corresponds to the frequency of the Earth's trajectory around the sun.

And it follows that the appropriate scent could only be that of the lemon. The clear freshness of the lemon's aroma stimulates the natural sphere of vibrations – the citric acid cycle – within our liver. This cycle is vital to our entire metabolism, which provides our body with energy.

On the subtle plane it opens up the solar chakra and thereby allows access to our own subconscious – our primal knowledge.

The harmonious interaction of all stimulating factors on the solar chakra will eventually make existential fears dissolve, and thusly we can – as stated in an old saying – "...make human beings into gods, as one takes away their fears."

In this ideal state we are again in contact with the divine spark within us and so have regained our link with the Divine, whose impuls reaches us through our receiver, the THROAT CHAKRA.

The Throat Chakra

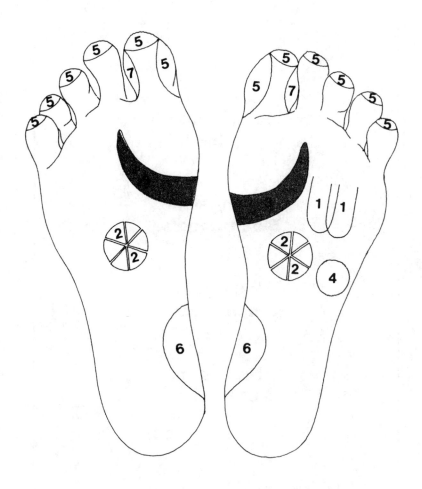

"Not what enters the human being from the outside sullies it, but instead that, which comes out of it from inside."

Healing color:
Blue

Healing stone:
Blue turquoise

Healing tone:
Moon tone

Healing oil:
Lavender oil

Throat Chakra Massage

These words of the Bible fittingly describe the function of our throat chakra. Our receiving of anything is completely neutral when it occurs. What we do with it, however, we are responsible for.

Goethe, the great literary figure and esoteric, wrote in Faust: "Firstly we are free, secondly we are slaves." Which is to say that we are completely free in regard to thoughts and other information – vibrations – that we let enter us, but then we are also bound – to the consequences!

Being responsible for oneself appears to be an all but unsolvable problem for a lot of people beset by blockades in their throat chakra. These may then manifest as physical symptoms, such as difficulty swallowing, chronic hoarseness, problems of the thyroid gland, tonsilitis and, in the simplest of cases, spotted skin due to a hectic state.

Our respiration organs, too, are connected with the throat chakra on the subtle plane, as through them we take on air and with it life energy. Therefore we may find asthmatics also suffering from blockades of the throat chakra.

The massage technique consists of gently

switching from the solar plexus point to the terminal nerve point of the thyroid gland and initially massaging this on the left foot for two minutes, followed by the same procedure with the right foot. Do not forget to have your patient visualize the color blue, the healing color of the throat chakra.

While doing this, let the patient take up spiritual contact with the element of water, in any configuration whatsoever. This works a profound purefication, in the course of which all "unclean" thoughts, all of the ballast and suffering and any pain being experienced can be "washed away".

Once the mental sphere is purefied by the harmonization of the throat chakra, the two blue-colored elements in nature, water and the heavens, will melt into one another at the horizon of their visualization.

When this harmony is reached we are "free" at the physical as well as the spiritual level. We then feel ourselves as unlimited as the horizon, no matter what our situation in the Here and Now may be.

The healing stone of the throat chakra is the blue turquoise. As my work with patients has shown me, it radiates the greatest power for this energy center. That is why you should place a blue turquoise on the area of the thyroid gland during the massage.

The moon tone completes the vibrations of

the energy center with this stone. It corresponds to the frequency of the moon, which determines the flow of the tides, but also the cycles of human beings.

Quite a few people will instictively visualize an intensely blue field of lavender, like the ones one can experience with one's entire being in the Provence region of France in the summer. And that is the fragrance that vibrates in harmony with our throat chakra. So when treating disturbances of the throat chakra, apply drops of lavender oil the way previously described.

If, while you are massaging for a blocked throat chakra, the patient should develop difficulty swallowing or a "lump in the throat" sets in, have him or her swallow vigorously a few times and this feeling will quickly fade away.

In the harmony with the Divine, which we can achieve via the throat chakra, our self-confidence will grow, as will our our faith, which in the body is located in the SACRAL CHAKRA.

The Sacral Chakra

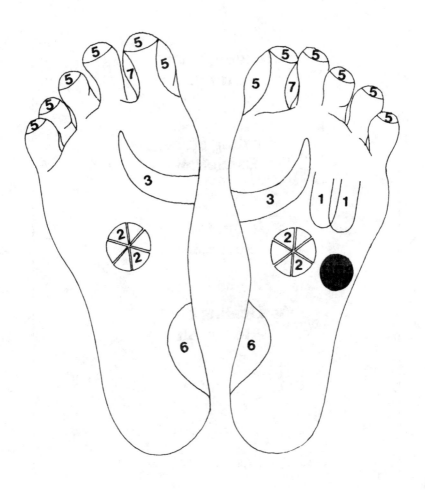

"All Healing lies in Faith..."

Healing color:
Orange

Healing stone:
Carnelian

Healing tone:
Sun tone

Healing oil:
Neroli oil

Sacral Chakra Massage

Healing can only be worked when patient and therapist believe in it.

This realization also shows us the far-reaching significance of the sacral chakra for well-being through mental power.

The reflexology zone for the sacral chakra is located on the left foot, and is identical with the terminal nerve point of the spleen. Again, we massage for the duration of two minutes using rotating pressure. Frequently the patient will immediately feel an intense sensation of warmth in the area of the upper abdomen.

At the same time we suggest the visualization of the color orange, in which the patient should immerse the spleen in the left side of the body beneath the costal arch.

Symptoms of sickness resulting from disturbances of the sacral chakra usually do not manifest in forms that are easily identified and classified, as with the other chakras. The best example of this is diabetes, an insidious metabolic disease of the pancreas, which is also governed by the sacral chakra.

The patients themselves destroy their joy, the "sweetness" of life, and this effects the entire organism.

The same connection can be found in the case of leukemia, whose effects are systemic yet most severely befall the spleen, the organ mainly involved with our blood. Here again we are confronted with a state of illness in which the emotional themes of primal trust (faith) are unsolved.

Such diffuse conditions of sickness can only be influenced by a very powerful healing stone: the orange-red carnelian. It enhances the blood circulation within the spleen and on the subtle plane influences the sacral chakra. In this way self-healing forces are activated.

The tone of the sun flows into the sphere of vibration of the sacral chakra like an orange-golden rain, and amplifies its power.

Primal knowledge and faith draw from the same source of energy. This explains the effect of the sun tone on the solar plexus and the sacral chakra.

And the scent vibrations of neroli oil, derived from orange blossoms, fits into this constellation with its freshness and warmth. The color sequence of the bright yellow midday sun becoming the orange-red sphere of the evening sky symbolizes the scope of the close connection between the solar chakra and the sacral chakra. In the union of primal knowledge at the horizon, the melting together of Earth and sky, and in faith in the sun ever rising the next morning, our human existence is also mirrored in the chakras.

The belief in reincarnation therefore is also deeply rooted in our subtle sphere.

When one has completely activated this chakra, one has found access to an immense source of strength: faith.

In this faith also rests our mental power, which can work externally through our transmitter, the INNER EYE CHAKRA.

The Inner Eye Chakra

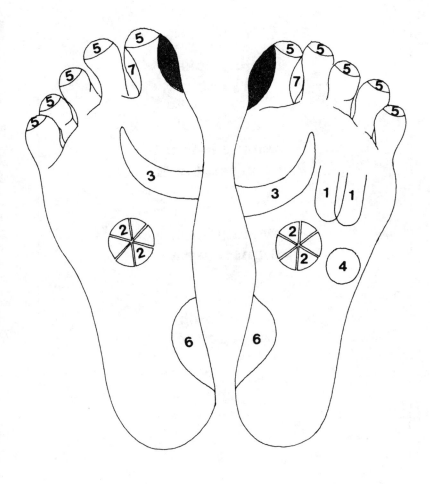

"Thoughts are unhindered..."

Healing color:
Violet

Healing stone:
Rock crystal point

Healing tone:
Jupiter tone

Healing oil:
Lavender oil

Inner Eye Chakra Massage

Has it ever happened to you that you were intensely thinking about someone when suddenly the phone rang and precisely that person called you? That is only one form of mental power.

I am convinced that thoughts really can move mountains, and since I know what powers they have, I am well aware of my responsibility for every one of my thoughts.

Everything one thinks manifests in one form or another – whether positive or negative! We decide what we create.

Our environment is the visible expression of the negativeness of our thinking: dying forests, polluted rivers, poisoned air... All of that is not outside of us, its root lie in us, and therefore we all are responsible for the condition our environment is in.

And what about our own body? If I am constantly programming the cells of my body negatively, for instance with fear, envy, hate, even self-hate and anger, need I be surprised if they degenerate, if they turn out like my thoughts? Cause and effect are obvious in these depictions.

In their origin thoughts are completely neutral. Only through the emotions we attach to them – our "judging" – do we lend them positive or negative power, and for these effects we are fully responsible.

Epilepsy is the illness that has the most appropriate symbolic value for the inner eye chakra. Prior to every major seizure the patient experiences an "aura", the medical term for the sensory phenomenon that includes colors, smells and sounds, and signals the patient that he or she is about to "drop out" into a different realm. The seizure itself is marked by cramp-like convulsions of the entire body. Apparently, uncoordinated impulses are sent at the physical as well as subtle level.

On the foot we find the massage point for the inner eye chakra in the area of the sinus at the tip of the big toe. We alternate massaging these areas with rotating pressure on each foot for two minutes.

Violet is the highest spiritual color, as ultraviolet has the greatest range within the spectrum. This predestinates it to be the healing color for our sending center. The patient should in his or her visualization let violet flow into his frontal sinus, so that it is completely lined with it.

The power of our sending center is amplified by rock crystal. It is the healing mineral with the most direct effect. Particularly suitable are rock crystal points, and they are placed onto the area of the inner eye pointing upward along the body towards the crown chakra. Not the color of a stone but rather its vibrations determine its optimal healing effects on the chakra.

The Jupiter tone enhances the development towards the highest spiritual level, just as the planet Jupiter in astrology points to the fact that a person living under this sign may find ways to a high degree of spirituality. Its vibrations are the perfect augmentation of the inner eye.

Sender and receiver must share the same frequency, or no communication will be possible. This explains the fact that lavender emits the scent-vibration connected with the throat chakra and the inner eye chakra. Apply the oil prior to massaging the patient as previously described.

The inner eye chakra is the only one not bound to an organ or part of the body; it is universal. Disturbances at the inner eye therefore do not lead to a specific physical symptom, but instead effect the organism as a whole. Its coordination suffers.

The vibratory energy of the inner eye does not need to materialize: the spirit works unhampered by limits of time and space, and it alone remains after we leave our physical body. That is the spiritual evolution into the subconscious:

"...yet, thoughts are unhindered...",

and with precisely this thought in mind we
now immerse ourselves in the power sphere
of the ROOT CHAKRA.

The Root Chakra

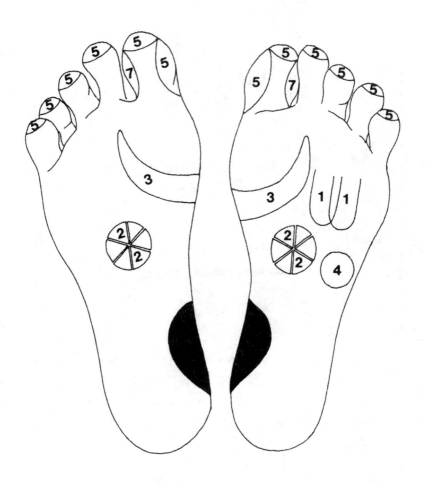

"Thus spoke Zeus: 'Come, let us go, my root lusts, let us create a hero...'"

Healing color:
Red

Healing stone:
Jasper

Healing tone:
Shiva-Shakti tone

Healing oil:
Lotus oil

Root Chakra Massage

The seat of our most elementary vital force is the root chakra, located at the lower end of the spinal column. It influences all of our sex organs and our drive to procreate. It harbors our "lust" for life.

Much has been said and written about it. How much poetry, how many works of art and songs have come forth from this activated source of power. In this manner sexual energy is transformed and becomes spiritual, and that is the profoundest reason for existence.

The point is not to suffer in renunciation and self-castigation, but it will also not suffice to manifest this energy on a purely physical level. Only at the peak of the union between two people can we connect with the universal forces on a plane beyond our physical state, even if only for a few moments. And are we not all seeking the lasting transformation of our strongest power, our vital energy, into spiritual growth?

But how often is this quest in vain and the cause of various physical ailments, such as interruptions of the cycle, frigidity, impotence or tumor diseases. Unrealized or misguided sexual energy will also frequently manifest as migraine headaches or as remarkably frequent bladder trouble.

By applying a Chakra Energy Massage we can positively influence and harmonize the region of the sacrum via the feet and thereby eliminate numerous blockades. Therefore massage these terminal nerve points for the base of the spine consecutively on both feet for two minutes each.

Infrared has the shortest wave length within the spectrum, but at the same time a considerable heating effect. The healing color red for the root chakra also generates a great deal of warmth, which may be clearly felt with the hands. It is therefore beneficial to have the effects of this color be mentally included in cases of blockades of the lowest chakra.

If the person you are treating shows a pronounced blockade within this energy center, visualizing red will most likely present considerable difficulties. You can support the patient's efforts, however, by suggesting mental images to concentrate on, such as dark red roses. You will see that once the blockade begins to disappear the patient will no longer require your support in order to visualize color.

Yet there are numerous people who constantly "see red", whose root chakra is highly active and finds no release, people that are unable to live out their sexuality. They, too, will experience balancing, harmonizing effects from the Chakra Energy Massage.

For the supplementary mineral therapy in the root chakra I achieve my best results using red jasper. There are other stones that may also increase and accelerate the development of spirituality within this center, but I have observed genuine healing effects solely with jasper. Place the stone onto the patient's abdomen in the area of the pubic bone. The jasper will radiate deeply, all the way to the seat of the chakra.

The primal tone that works harmonizingly here is the so-called Shiva-Shakti tone, a combination of the sun and moon tones as well as those of the solar, sacral and throat chakras. The reason for combining all of these frequncies is that the entire abdominal region becomes receptive and thusly trust and devotion towards the partner can set in.

The fragrance capable of additionally increasing these emotions on the physical as well as subtle plane is that of the lotus blossom. The art of love matured to perfection in the East in a very early age, and so it is this cultural sphere that gives us the plant whose vibrations make it possible for us to open the root chakra and let it spiral up and transform itself into the CROWN CHAKRA.

The Crown Chakra

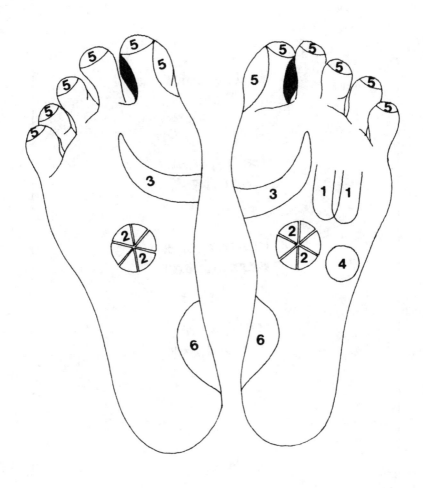

*"...and the Spirit of God
hovered above them."*

Healing color:
Gold

Healing stone:
Amethyst

Healing tone:
Karuna tone

Healing oil:
"Devotion"

The Crown Chakra

Many artists depicted the phenomenon of Whitsuntide visually as minute flames appearing above the heads of the apostles, and I find this to be an ingenious way of symbolizing enlightenment, the opening of the crown chakra.

The halo, too, is nothing other than a glow of the perfectly opened energy field reaching all the way into the causal realm.

We are all born with a skull not completely closed at the crown, the fontanels being open. In other words, with a physical expression of our crown chakra. As long as this has not closed, which takes place at about the age of three, we are in direct contact with the cosmos. Up until that time we are wise.

Wisdom has its seat in our crown chakra and we must open this in order to transform knowledge accumulating in the solar plexus into a state of wisdom. In this, small children are ahead of us adults.

The phenomenon of headache manifesting like a band around the upper head is quite simply explainable as a congestion of energy within the crown chakra. Problems of the pituitary gland can be traced back to blockades of this kind. As this gland is the control organ and regulator of all hormonal as well as emotionally influenced processes of the body, disharmonies in the area of the uppermost chakra affect all elemental life processes as well as the entire subtle plane. The reflexology zone of the crown chakra is the terminal nerve point of the pituitary gland on the inner side of the big toes. Therefore we massage these two reflexology zones consecutively for two minutes each using rotating pressure.

The most difficult task for the patient will probably be visualizing his or her pituitary gland surrounded by gold. Here, too, you should offer assistance by suggesting that the patient imagine the back of the head near the first cervical vertebra resting on a white gold pillow.

Gold is the healing color of the crown chakra, which is the point of departure for astral journeys.

Absolute harmony of vibration with our highest chakra is embodied by the diamond, that noblest of stones. But the healing stone for this chakra is the amethyst, whose vibrations are identical with those of the diamond. The diamond represents absolute purity while the amethyst is able to convey power. During the Chakra Energy Massage therefore place (as the final stone) an amethyst at the back of the patient's neck, directly at the junction with the skull.

The Karuna tone is the complete union of body, spirit and soul in audible form, and transcends into cosmic consciousness. Thus this tone is supreme perfection and opens up the highest center of energy. Just as this primal tone symbolizes the union of all frequencies, so the fragrance which influences the crown chakra ideally is a synthesis of 21 different scent essences.

At the close of the Chakra Energy Massage, after you have activated and harmonized all of the patient's energy centers, be sure to "spoil" him or her with the relaxation program described in detail on page 47.

My experience has shown that when very severe blockades are to be dealt with that are already manifesting physically, massages should be applied every third day, no sooner and no later.

Once the patient's state improves after a number of treatments, massages should be scheduled for every ninth day.

When the psyche's balance is again firmly established you may apply this massage occasionally at any time, but you do not necessarily have to.

You as therapist can also make use of the harmonizing effects of the Chakra Energy Massage. You are bound to find that this work with your patients costs you strength and energy and that you yourself must be in a state of harmony in order to be able to help others. So go ahead and apply what you have learned here to "recharge" yourself and to equalize the vibrations of your own chakras.

It is possible for you to massage your chakra points yourself, but it is more pleasant when someone does this for you.

Finally, I would like to share a realization with you which has become very important for me.

A Word of Advice in Closing

We receive cosmic information through our pituitary gland, our regulating center. From there the impulses are passed on to the thymus gland, which is connected to the heart chakra, so that the information can be experienced and lived by us through our emotions. We then transform it via the epiphysis to the transpersonal point, back to the universe.

And only if the thymus gland in connection with the heart chakra is in a state of perfect harmony, will we be in a position to transform everything streaming into us in the sense of UNIVERSAL LOVE.

Thus we fulfill the true purpose of our incarnation in this state of BEING.

Please regard this as a message from the spiritual world for your work with Chakra Energy Massage.

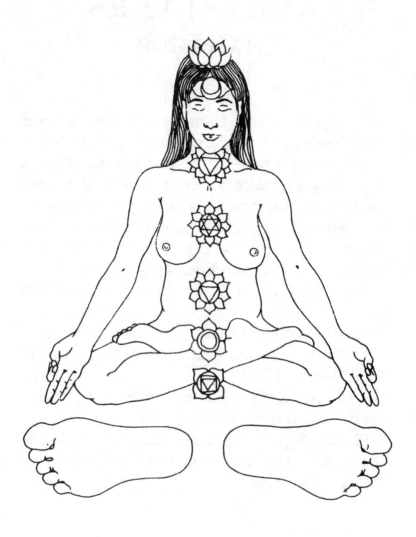

Table of the Chakras

Chakra	Healing Color	Healing Stone	Healing Tone	Healing Oil
Heart chakra	Pink	Rose quartz	Earth tone	Rose oil
Solar chakra	Yellow	Citrine	Sun tone	Lemon oil
Throat chakra	Blue	Blue turquoise	Moon tone	Lavender oil
Sacral chakra	Orange	Carnelian	Sun tone	Neroli oil
Inner eye chakra	Violet	Rock crystal	Jupiter tone	Lavender oil
Root chakra	Red	Jasper	Shiva-Shakti tone	Lotus oil
Crown chakra	Gold	Amethyst	Karuna tone	"Devotion"

ADDRESSES and SOURCES of SUPPLY
Fragrances, Gemstones, Herbs Books and Cassettes

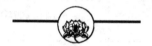

WHOLESALE

Contact with your business name,

resale number or practitioner license.

LOTUS LIGHT
Box 1008 CE
Silver Lake, WI 53170
Voice 414/889-8501 • Fax 414/889-8591

RETAIL

LOTUS FULFILLMENT SERVICE
33719 116th St, Box CE
Twin Lakes, WI 53181

Notes

Notes

Notes

Notes

CHAKRA ENERGY MASSAGE

By Marianne Uhl

$9.95; 128 pp.; paper; ISBN: 0-941524-83-3

Spiritual evolution into the subconscious through activation of the energy points of the feet.

This book introduces the concept of opening the subtle energy centers of the body through use of foot reflexology.

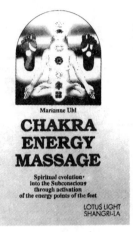

Marianne Uhl

CHAKRA ENERGY MASSAGE

Spiritual evolution into the Subconscious through activation of the energy points of the feet

LOTUS LIGHT
SHANGRI-LA

SECRETS OF PRECIOUS STONES

by Ursula Klinger Raatz

$9.95; 185 pp.; paper; ISBN: 0-941524-38-8

A guide to the activation of the seven human energy centers using gemstones, crystals and minerals.

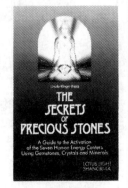

Ursula Klinger Raatz

THE SECRETS of PRECIOUS STONES

A Guide to the Activation of the Seven Human Energy Centers Using Gemstones, Crystals and Minerals

LOTUS LIGHT
SHANGRI-LA

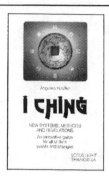
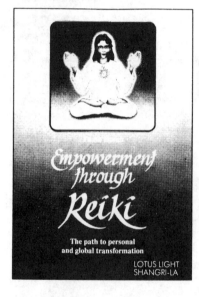
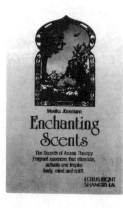

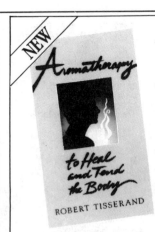
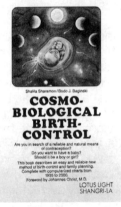
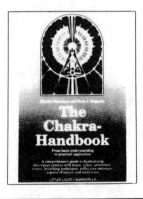

Angelika Höfler
I CHING
NEW SYSTEMS, METHODS
AND REVELATIONS
An innovative guide for all
of life's events and changes
190 Pages
ISBN 0-941424-37-X

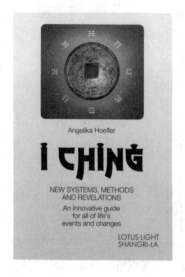

Angelika Hoefler

I CHING

NEW SYSTEMS, METHODS
AND REVELATIONS
An innovative guide
for all of life's
events and changes

LOTUS LIGHT
SHANGRI-LA

The I Ching – with new methods, new possibilities and new answers.

The author, herself actively interested in esoterics, studied characterology and applied as well as experimental psychology autodidactically, and has brought the eastern wisdom of the I Ching into poignant, contemporary language that includes glimpses of a knowing smile. In order to achieve exact answers, the hexagrams were divided into themes of inquiry, so that we can also receive concrete information about our own psychological make-up and condition, that of others and aspects of partnership. Each hexagram is accompanied by specific advice that is especially valuable in that it augments the partial as well as complete hexagram information, but can be applied independently of it. But the highlight of Angelika Hoefler's work is her development of a symbiosis of the I Ching and the Cabbala of Numbers, with which she has created a completely new system of cognition, of recognition and therewith practical help in life. We receive information, teachings, warnings, encouragement or advice, e. g. in questions of the right profession, place of education, living, work or vacation. Or in questions about the influence that certain persons or dates, agreements, names or titles to be decided on by us may have our success in life. Additionally, we gain clarity about where we stand in life–and this perhaps for the first time ever–what our functions and tasks are, where we belong and who belongs to us, and what the other person thinks about us.

Monika Jünemann
ENCHANTING SCENTS
The Secrets of Aroma Therapy.
Fragrant Essences that stimulate,
activate and inspire body, mind
and spirit
128 Pages
ISBN 0-941424-36-1

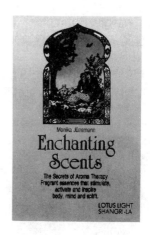

This book will carry you away to the world of exquisite, enchanting scents. Various fragrances effect our moods, may stimulate and excite us or bring us calmness and harmony, can bewitch and inspire, or even heal. Since ancient times essential oils and incenses have been employed in healing, for seduction and for religious rituals.

Today we are as captivated by the magic of lovely scents and as irresistably captivated by them as ever. The effects that essential oils have can vary greatly. This book particularly treats their subtle influences, but also presents and describes the plants from which they are obtained. *Enchanting Scents* beckons you to enter the realm of sensual experience, to journey into the world of fragrance through essences.

It is an invitation to employ personal, individual scents, to activate body and spirit, and to let your imagination soar. Here is a key that will open your senses to the limitless possibilities of benefitting from fragrances as stimulators, sources of energy and means of healing, or simply to let them broaden the scope of your own perception.

Ursula Klinger-Raatz
THE SECRETS OF PRECIOUS
STONES
A Guide to the Activation of the
Seven Human Energy Centers,
Using Gemstones, Crystals and
Minerals
128 Pages
ISBN 0-941424-38-8

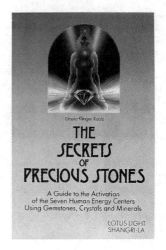

Ursula Klinger Raatz

THE
SECRETS
OF
PRECIOUS STONES

A Guide to the Activation
of the Seven Human Energy Centers
Using Gemstones, Crystals and Minerals

LOTUS LIGHT
SHANGRI-LA

Since time immemorial precious stones and crystals have been mysteriously fascinating for us human beings. Ursula Klinger Raatz describes the effects various stones have on our energy-body, which responds in a number of ways to the colors, qualities and uniqueness of minerals.

The author tells of her experiences with crystals and precious stones, describes the resonance they evoke, and explains how and why they are assigned to the different rainbow-colored energy centers of the human body.

This enables us to determine the healing vibrations of minerals right for us personally and to learn their practical application for the polarization of our energy centers, for healing using precious stones, and for entering into crystal meditation. Equally important, however, are the many impulses given for intuitive work with the secret powers inherent to the mineral world and particularly precious stones and crystals.